Body Weight

Educise 4 Kids

EDUCATION & EXERCISE FOR KIDS

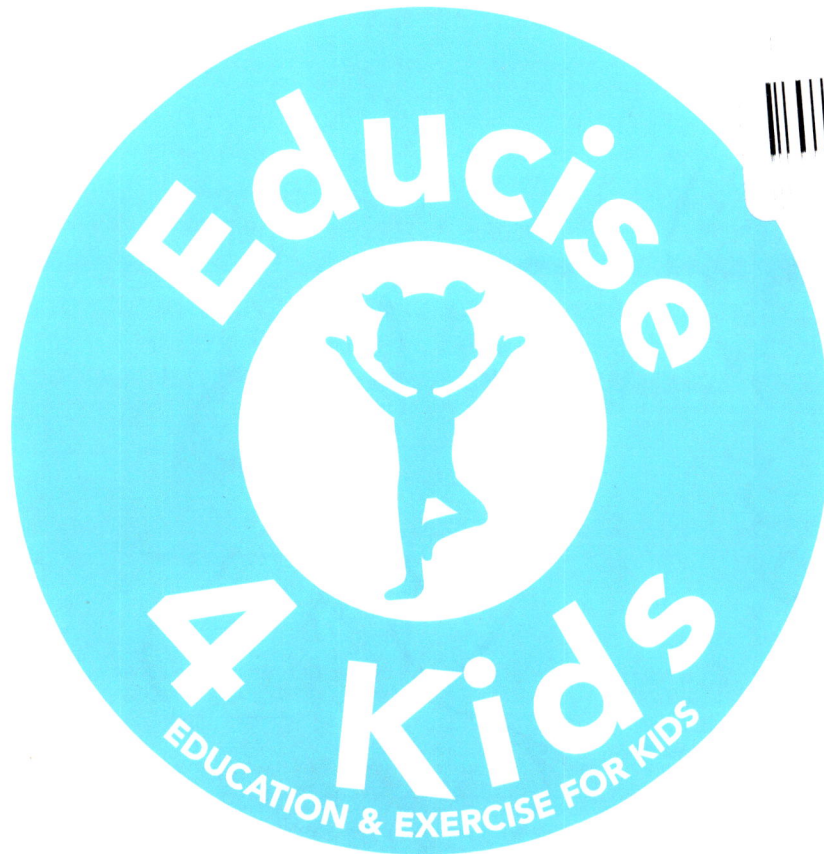

Created By
Priscilla Fauvette

Illustrated By
Bernard Fauvette

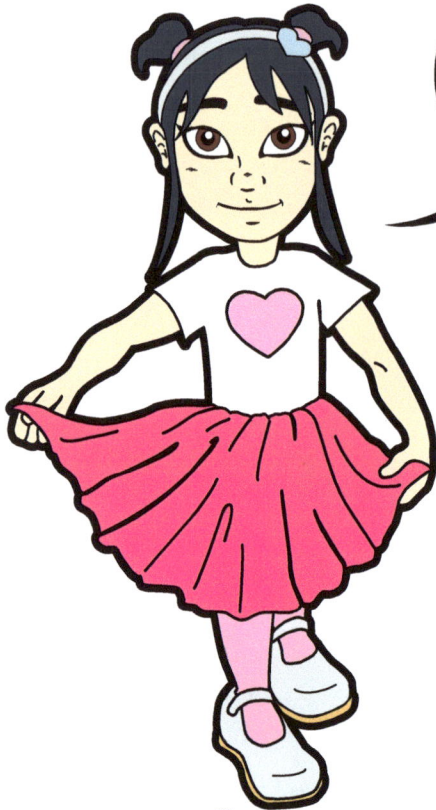

Lin

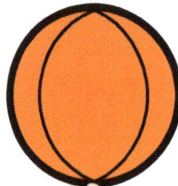

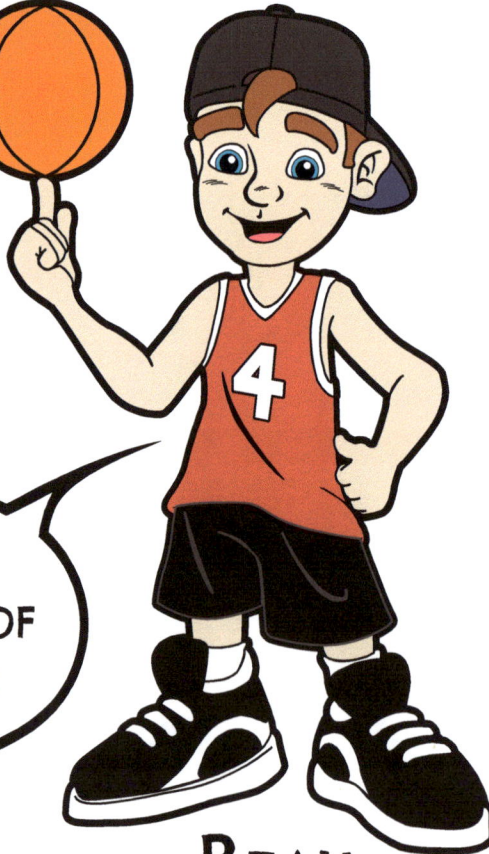

Beau

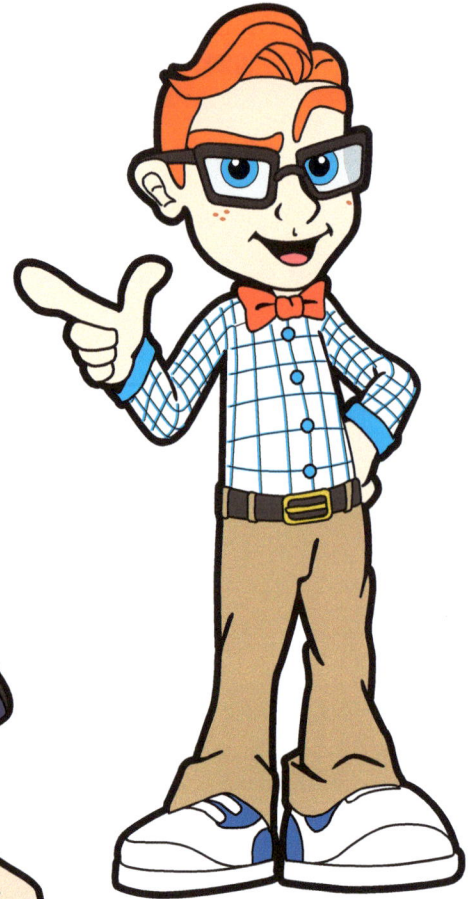

Caden

EAT PLENTY OF HEALTHY FOOD

LIMIT SCREEN TIME

MOVE YOUR BODY OFTEN

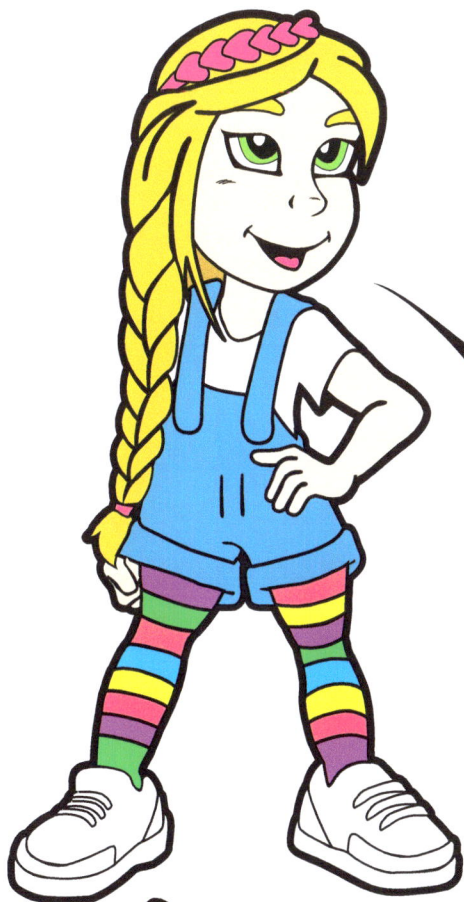

SOPHIE

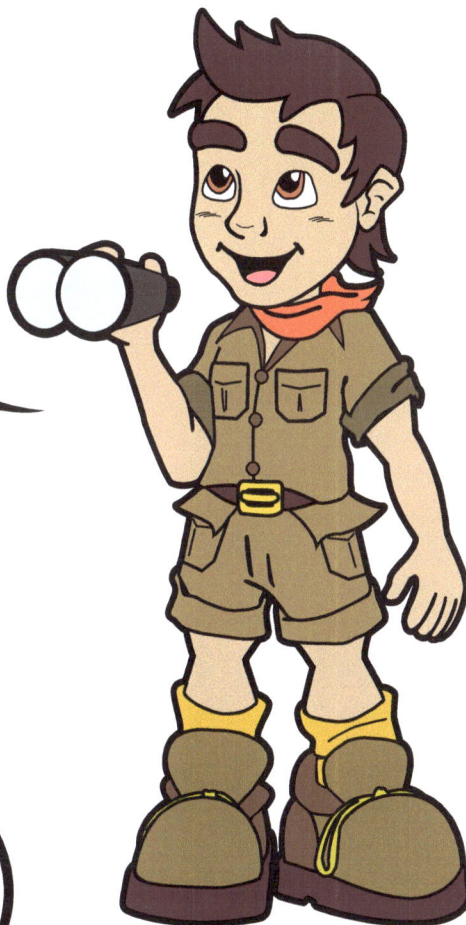

ZAC

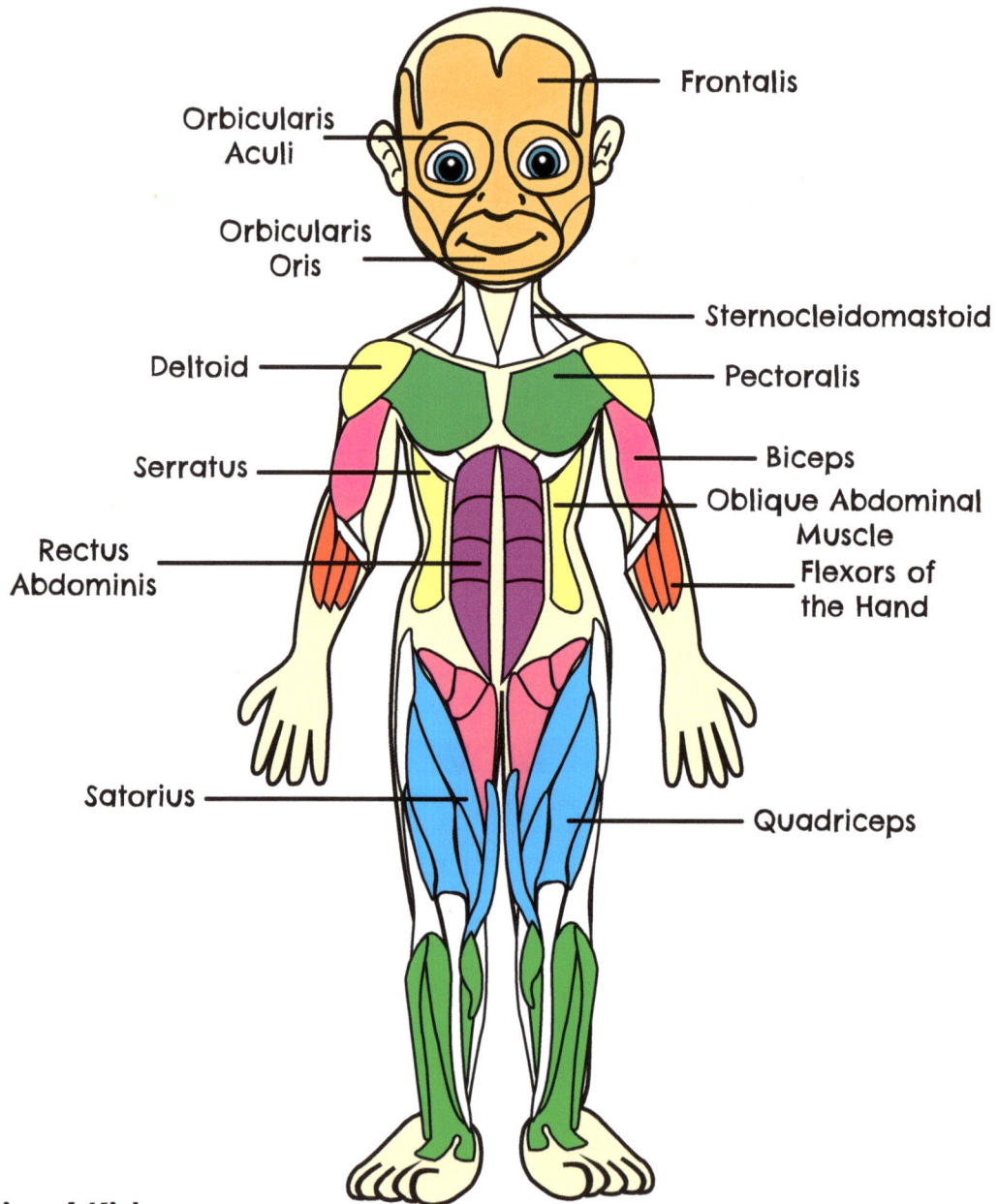

Anatomy

Frontalis

Orbicularis Aculi

Orbicularis Oris

Sternocleidomastoid

Deltoid

Pectoralis

Serratus

Biceps

Oblique Abdominal Muscle

Rectus Abdominis

Flexors of the Hand

Satorius

Quadriceps

Anatomy

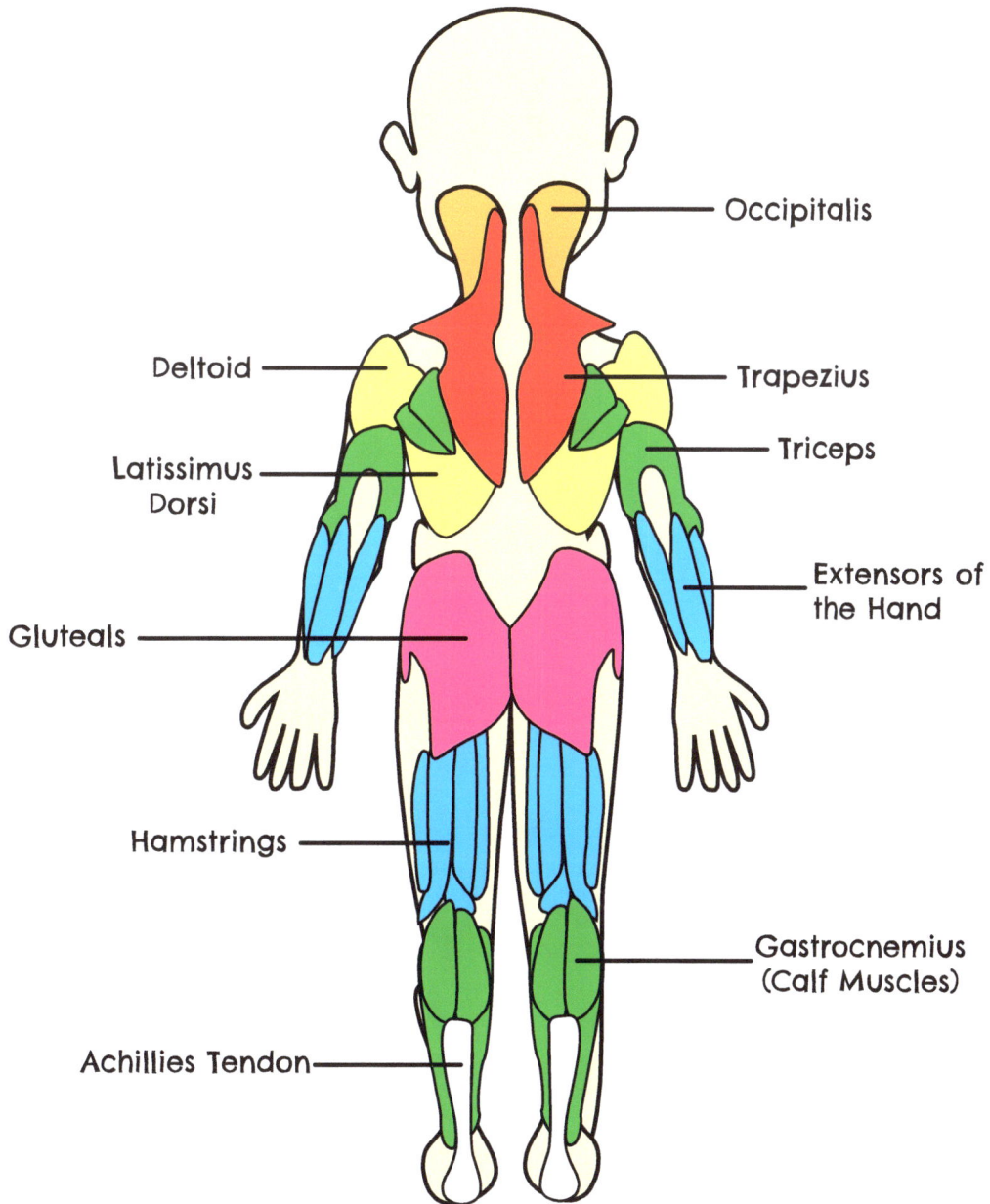

Occipitalis

Deltoid

Trapezius

Triceps

Latissimus Dorsi

Extensors of the Hand

Gluteals

Hamstrings

Gastrocnemius (Calf Muscles)

Achillies Tendon

Supermans

Lay your body on the floor

Straighten out your arms

Straighten out your legs and point your toes

Slowly lift your arms and your legs up together

Lower them back down again together

Can you do this 5 times?

1.

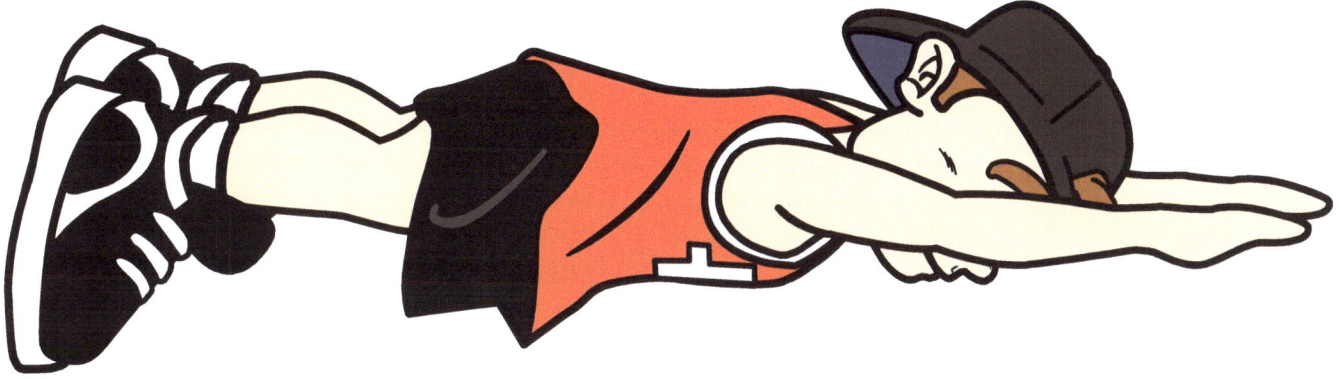

2.

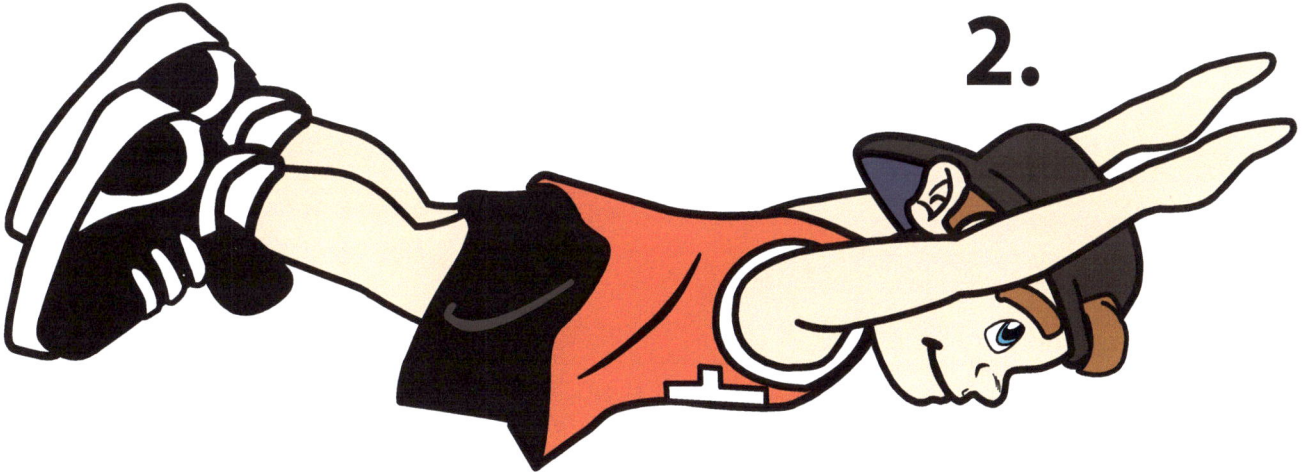

Bicycles

Lay down on the floor

Bend your knees and face them up

Place your hands behind your head

Slowly bring each elbow to touch

the opposite knee

Repeat this with each knee to elbow

Keep your stomach tight

Can you do this 5 times?

1.

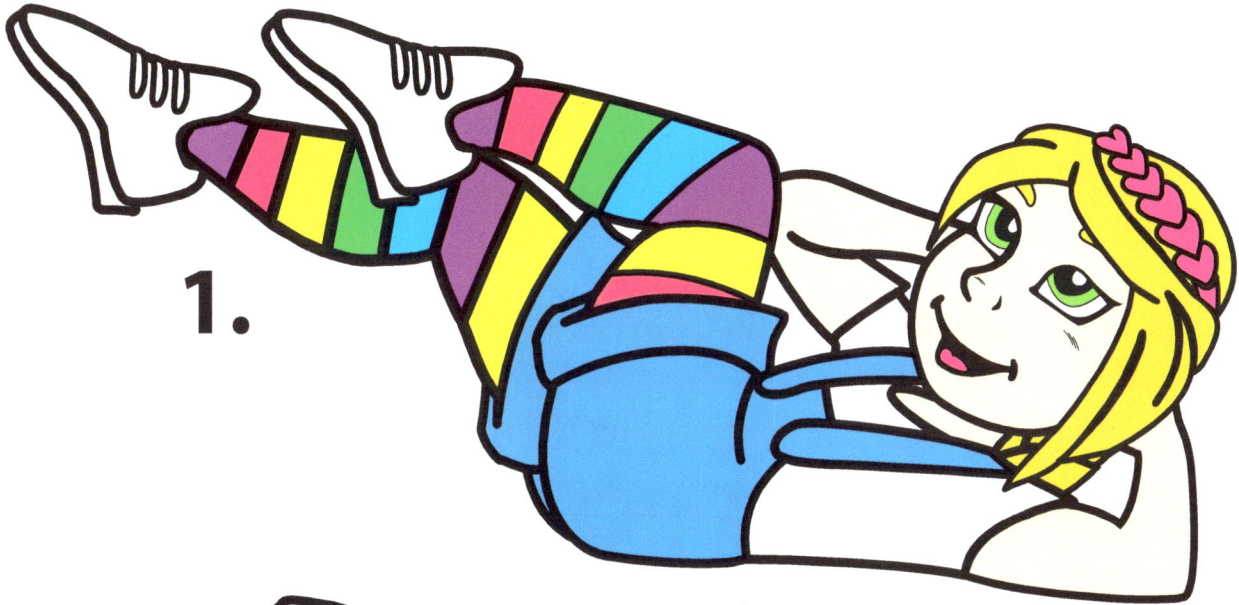

2.

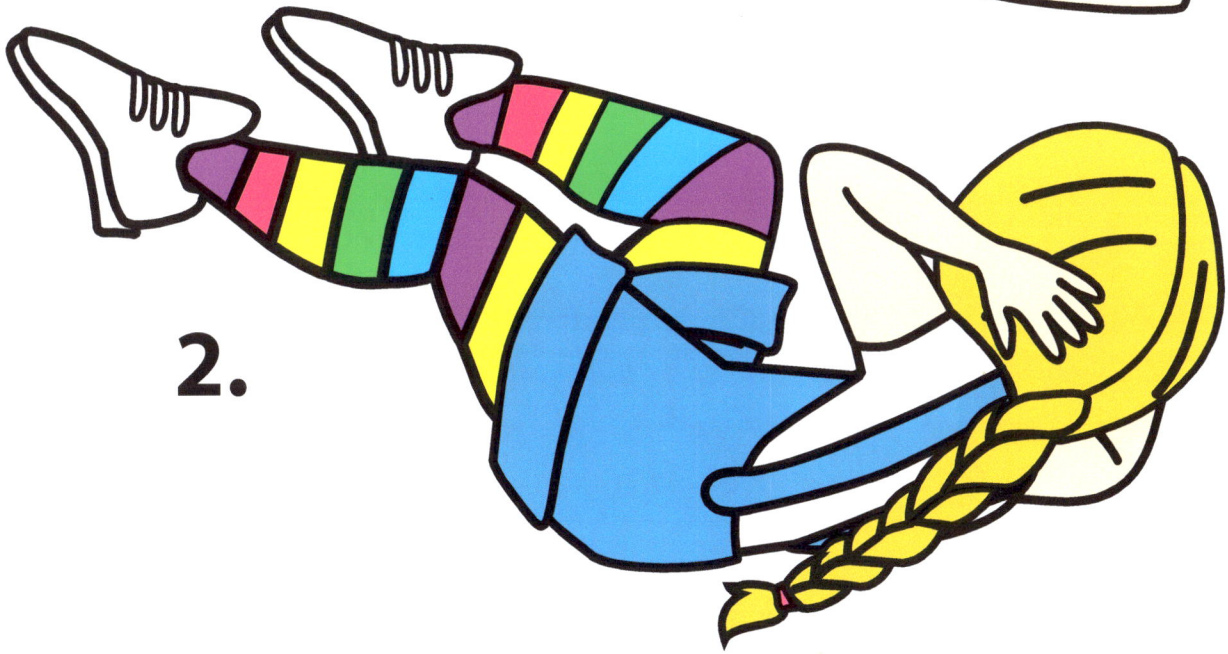

Tricep Dips

Sit on the floor

Bend your knees and face them up

Place your palms behind you on the floor

Slowly lift your body up

Straighten out your arms

Stay in this position

Slowly bend your elbows

Lower your body to the floor

Can you do this 5 times?

1.

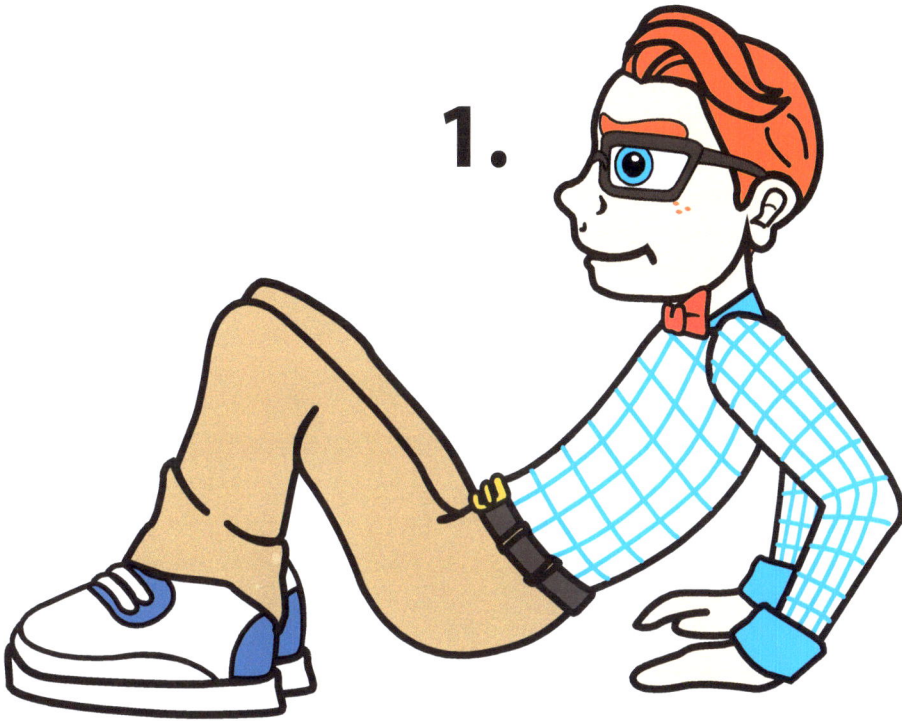

2.

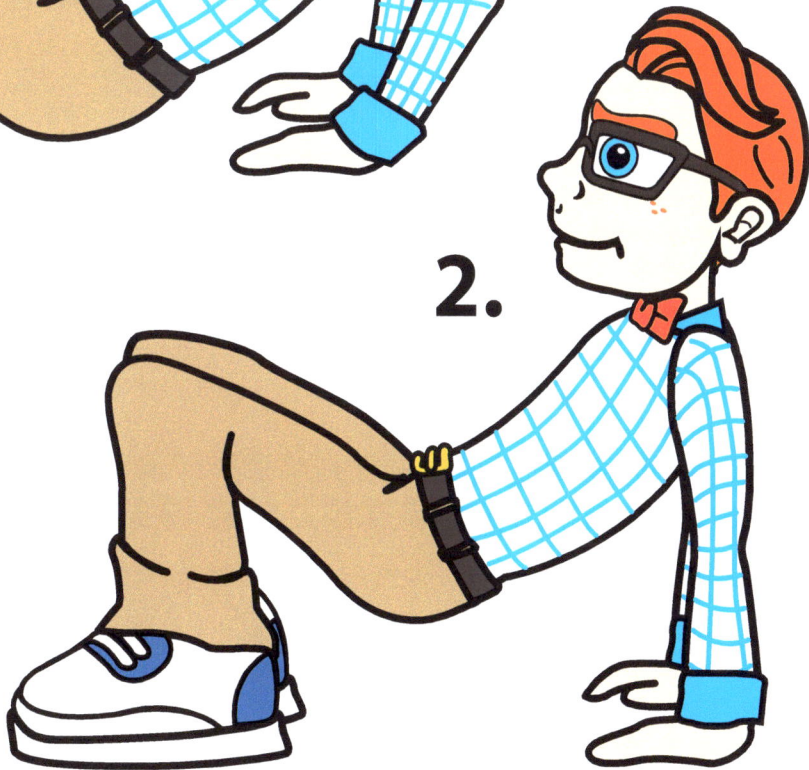

Arm Circles

Stand up straight

Raise your arms out to the side

Slowly circle your arms forward

Now slowly circle them backwards

Can you do this 5 times each way?

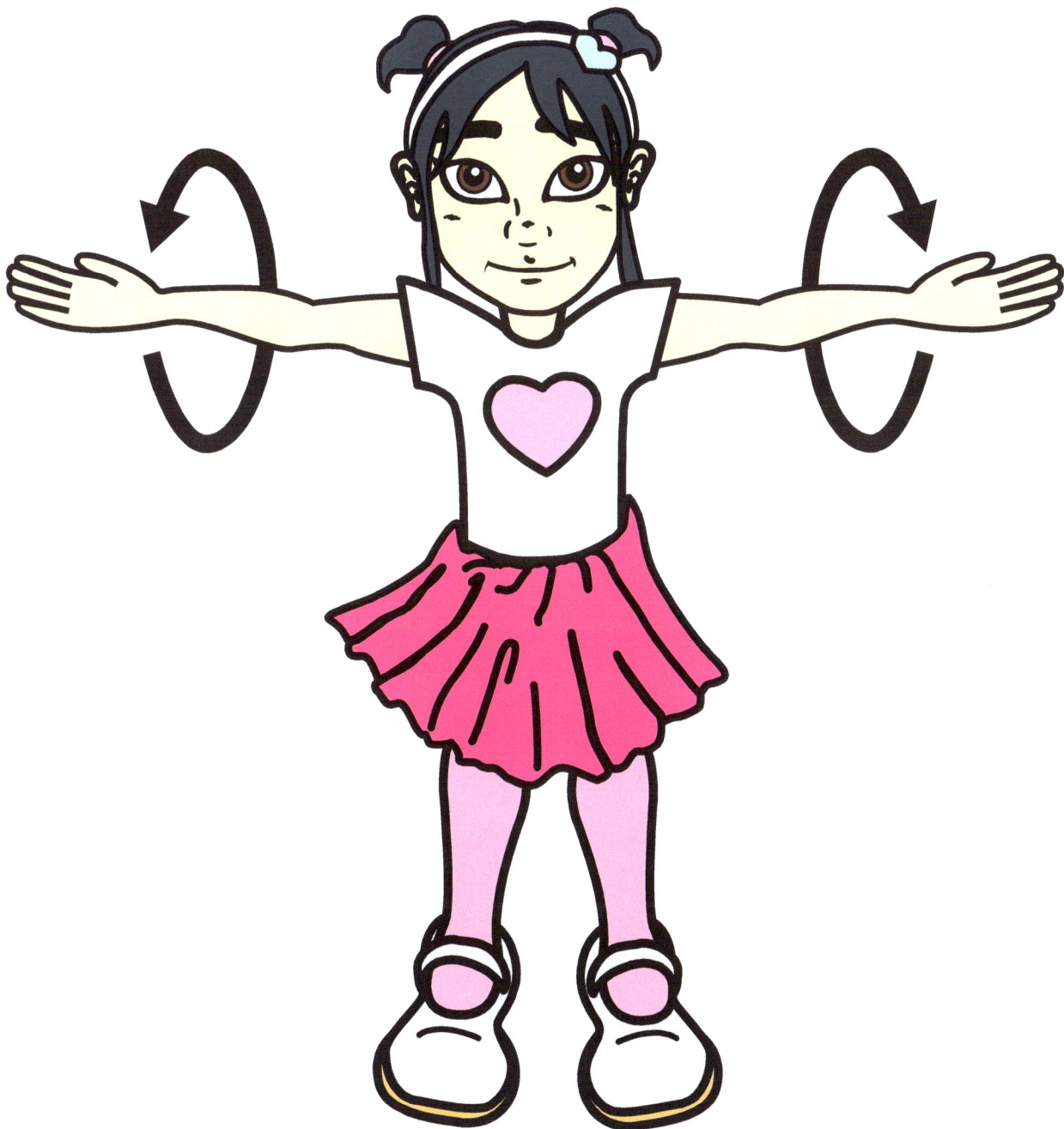

Lunges

Stand up straight

Take one step forward

Slowly lower your back leg

Keep your back straight

Now push yourself back up again

Can you do this 5 times on each side?

1.

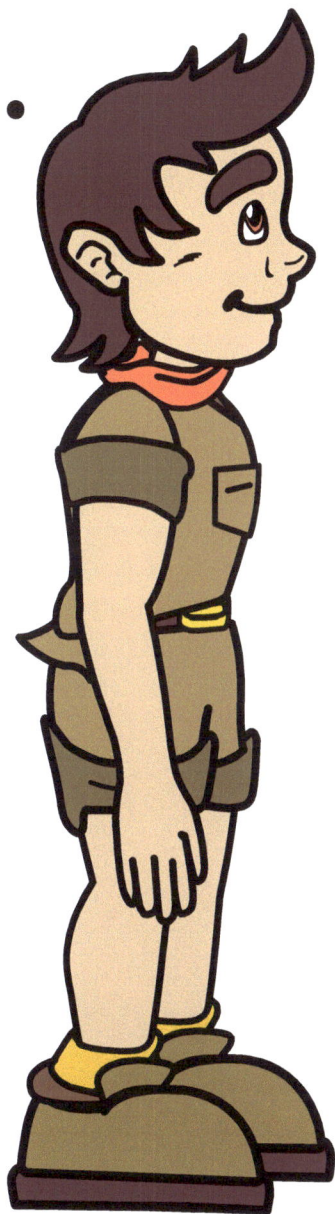

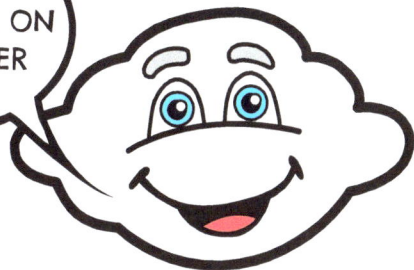

2.

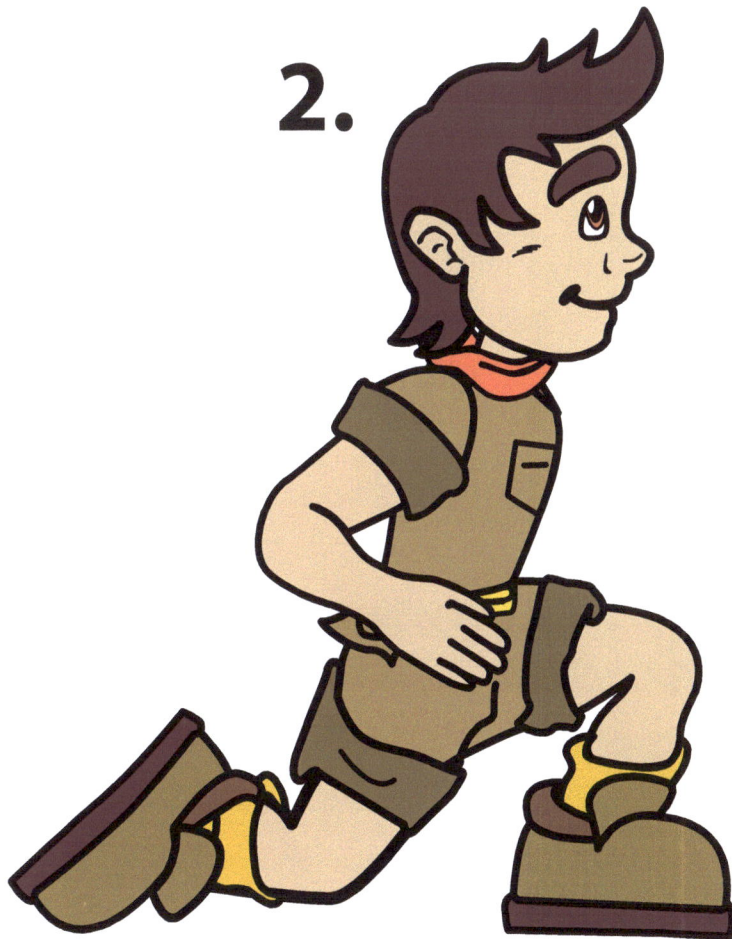

Push Ups

Lay flat on the floor
Place your hands beside your body
as wide as your shoulders
Push your whole body up
Keep your arms and back straight
Slowly lower your body back down
Can you do this 5 times?

1.

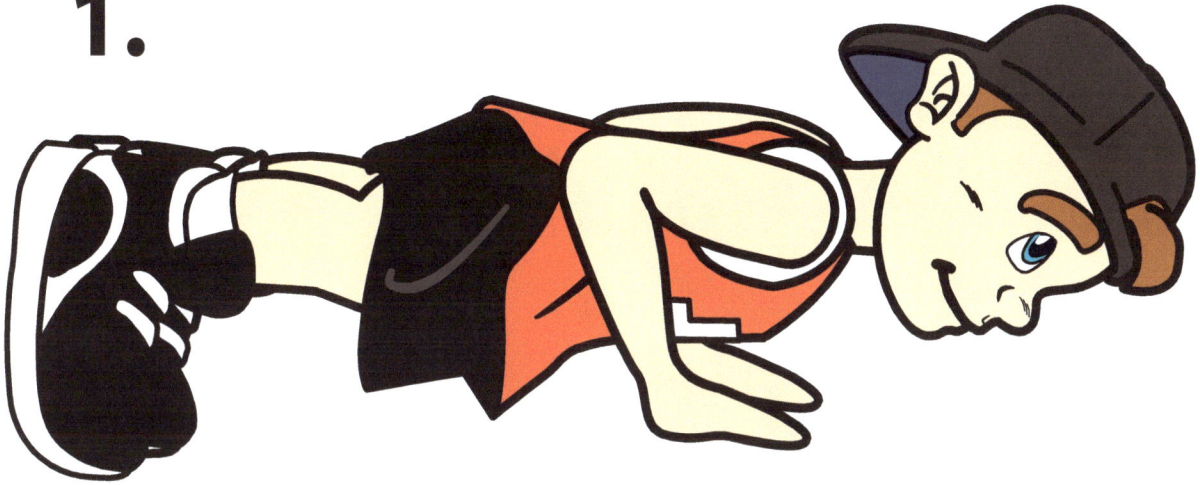

2.

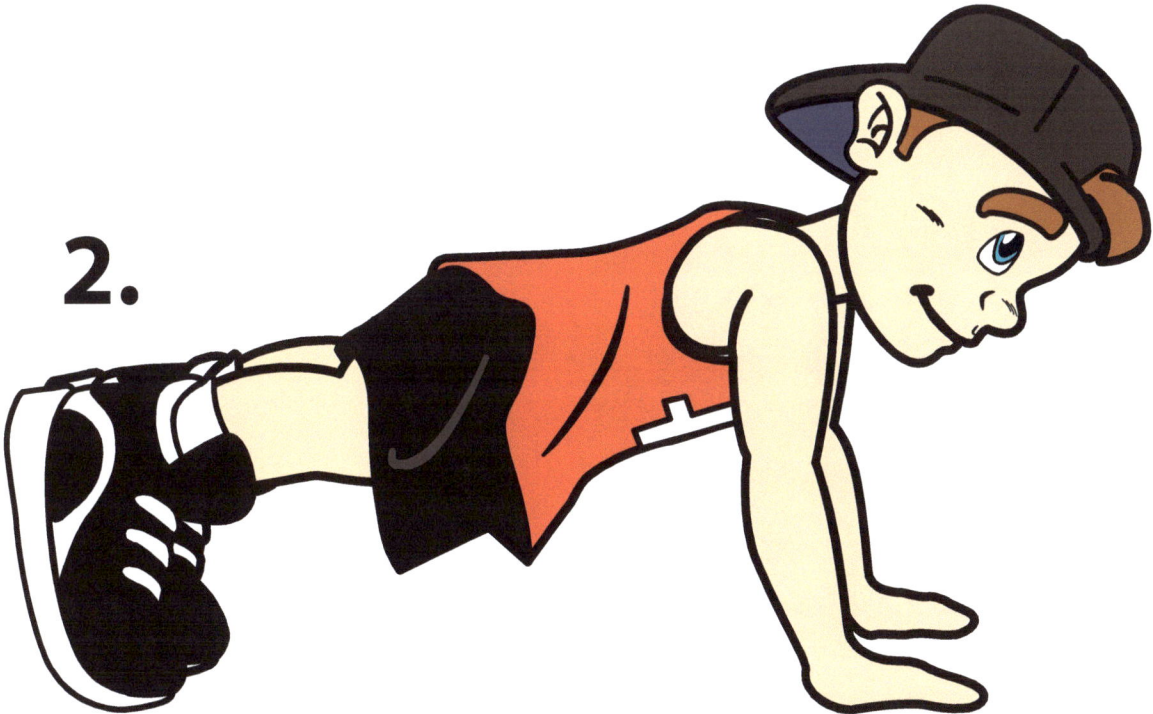

Heel Taps

Lay down on the floor

Bend your knees and face them up

Keeping your body mostly still reach out

with your hand and touch your ankle

Keep your stomach tight

Can you do this 5 times?

1.

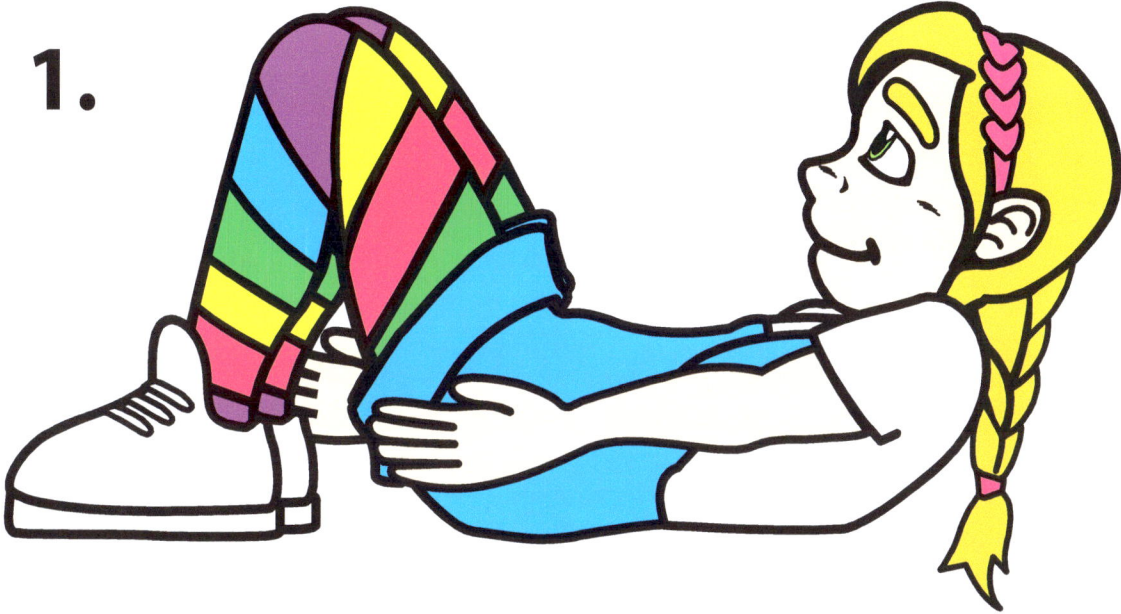

2.

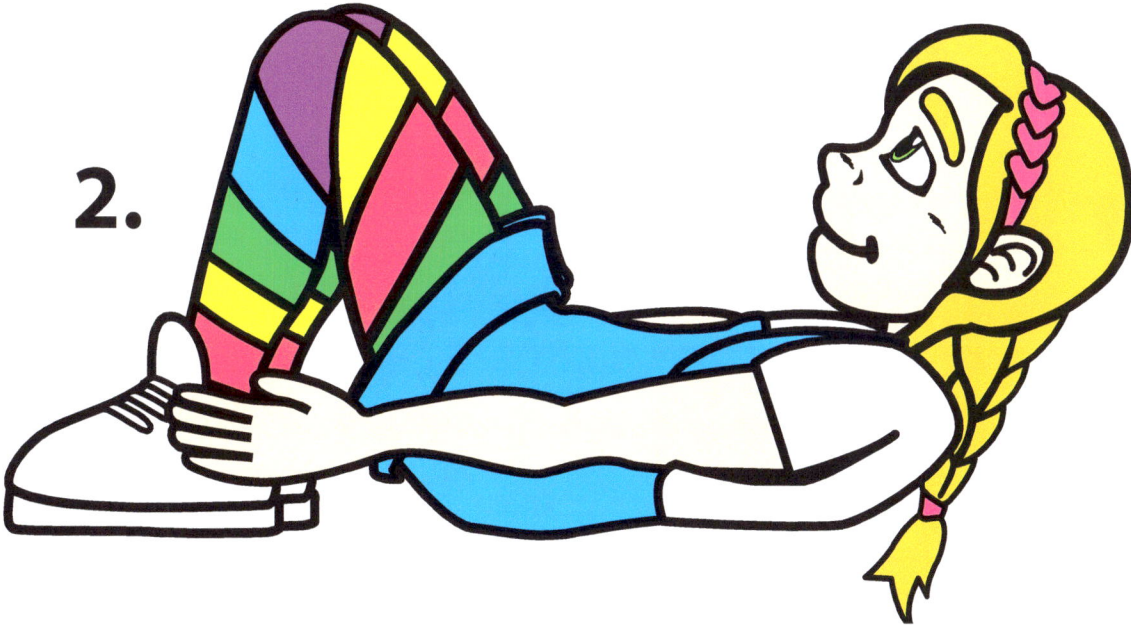

Wide Push Ups

Lay flat on the floor

Place your hands beside your body

as wide as you can

Push your whole body up

Keeps your arms and back straight

Slowly lower your body back down

Can you do this 5 times?

1.

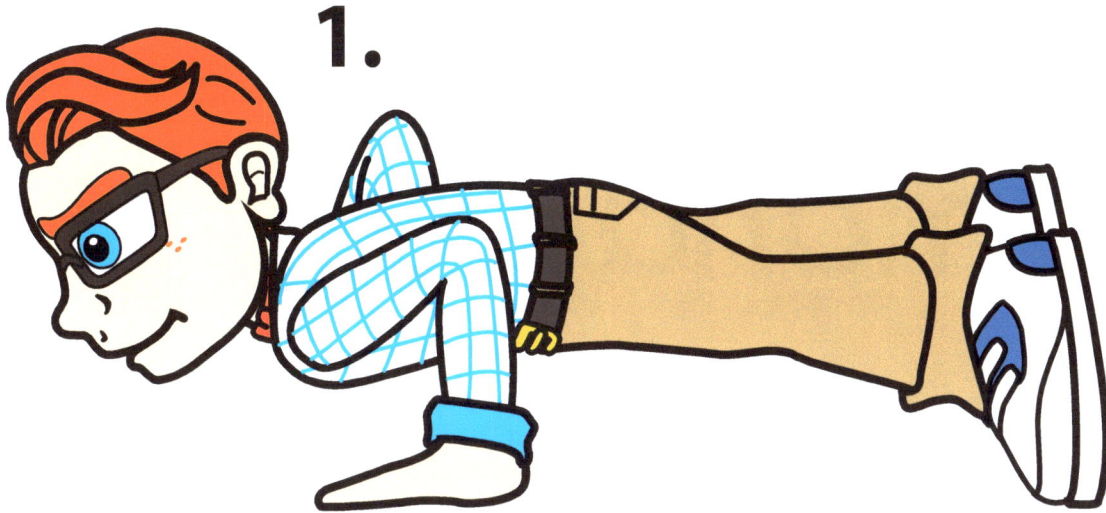

2.

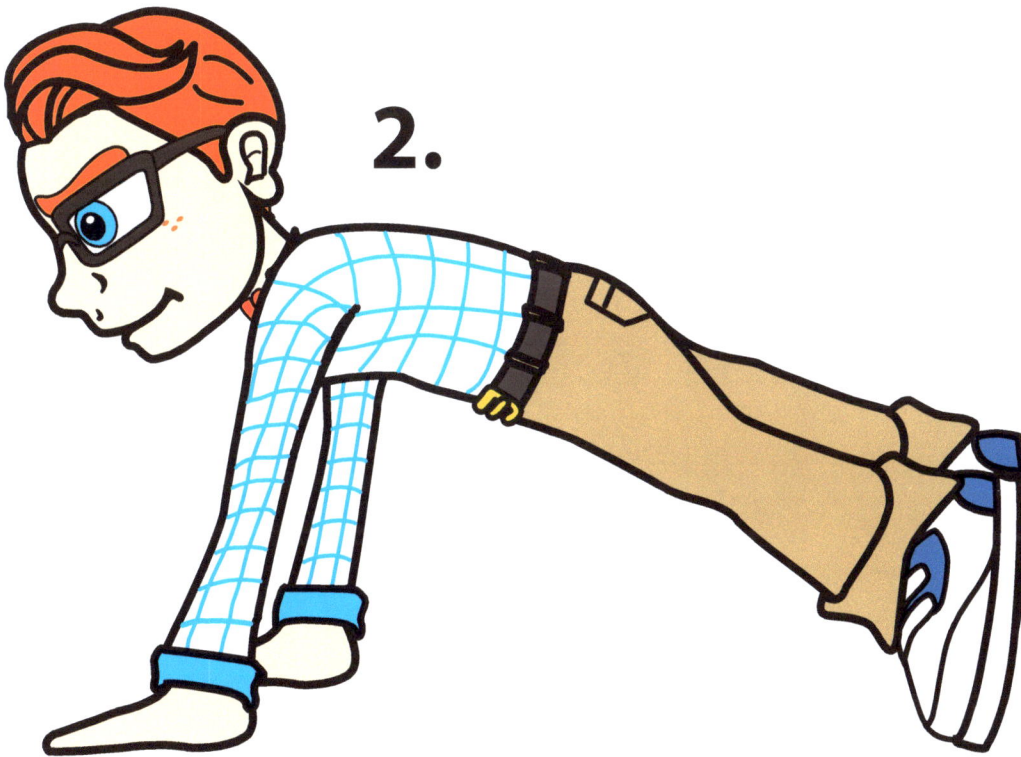

Diamond Push Ups

Lay your body on the floor
Place your hands underneath your chest
Shape your hands into a diamond
Push your body up until your arms are straight
Slowly lower your body down again
bending your elbows
Can you do this 5 times?

1.

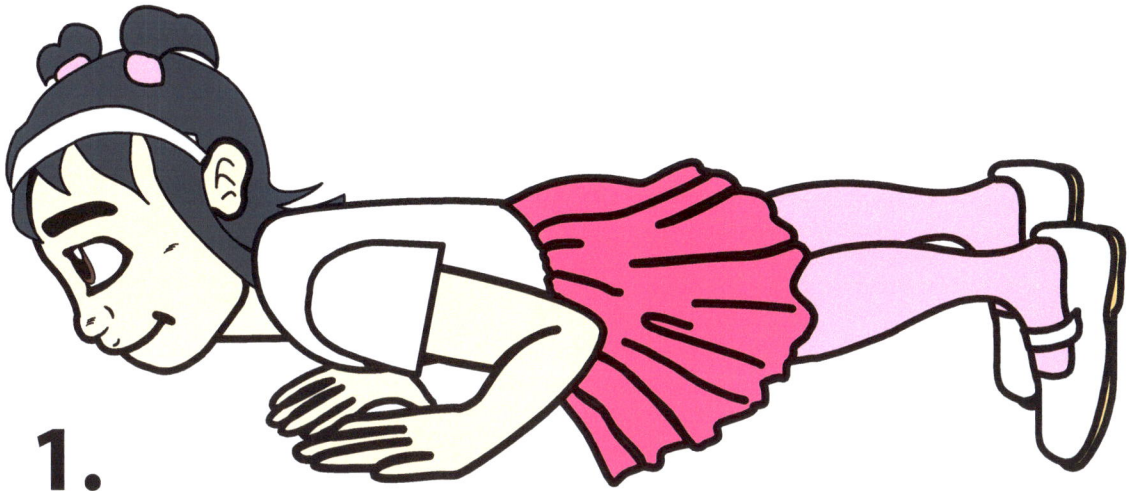

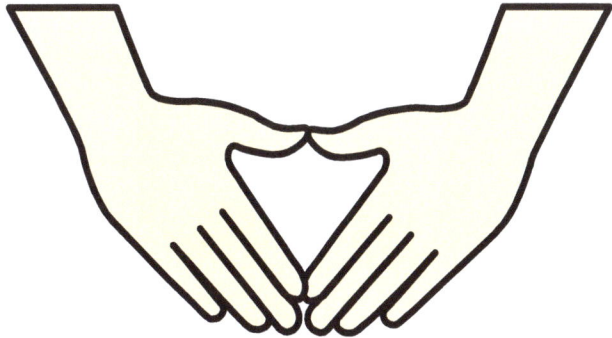

2.

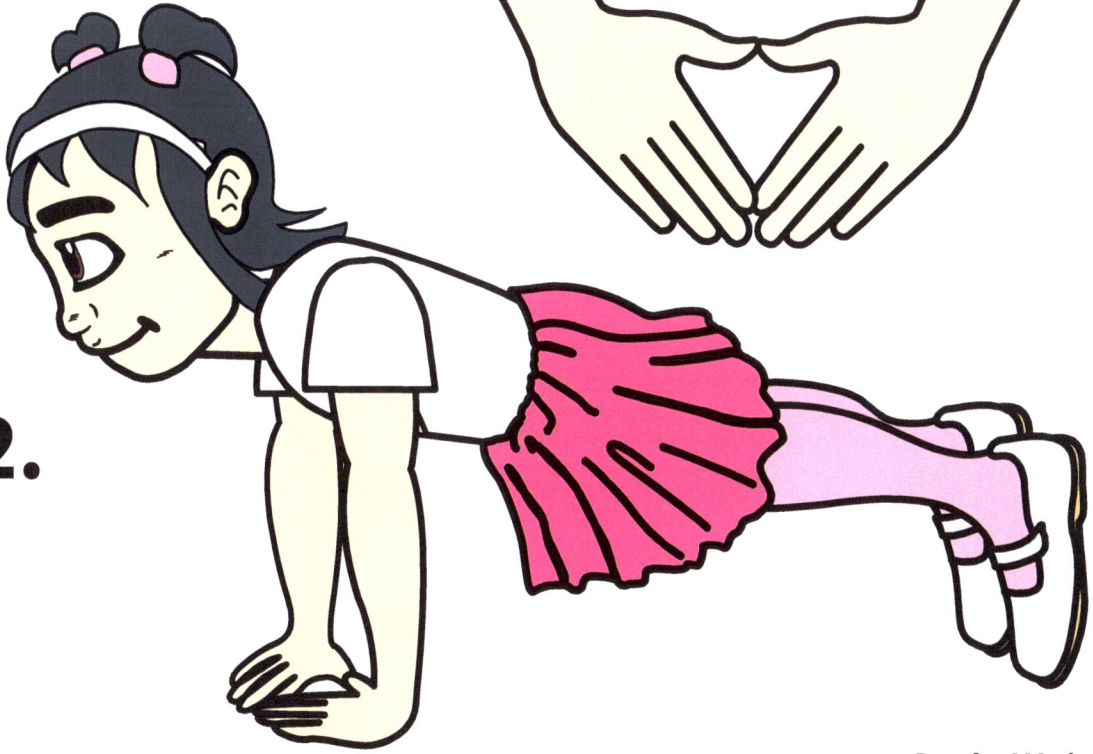

Crunches

Lay down on the floor

Bend your knees and face them up

Place your hands behind your head

Slowly lift yourself up and tighten

your stomach at the top

Lower yourself back down again to the floor

Can you do this 5 times?

1.

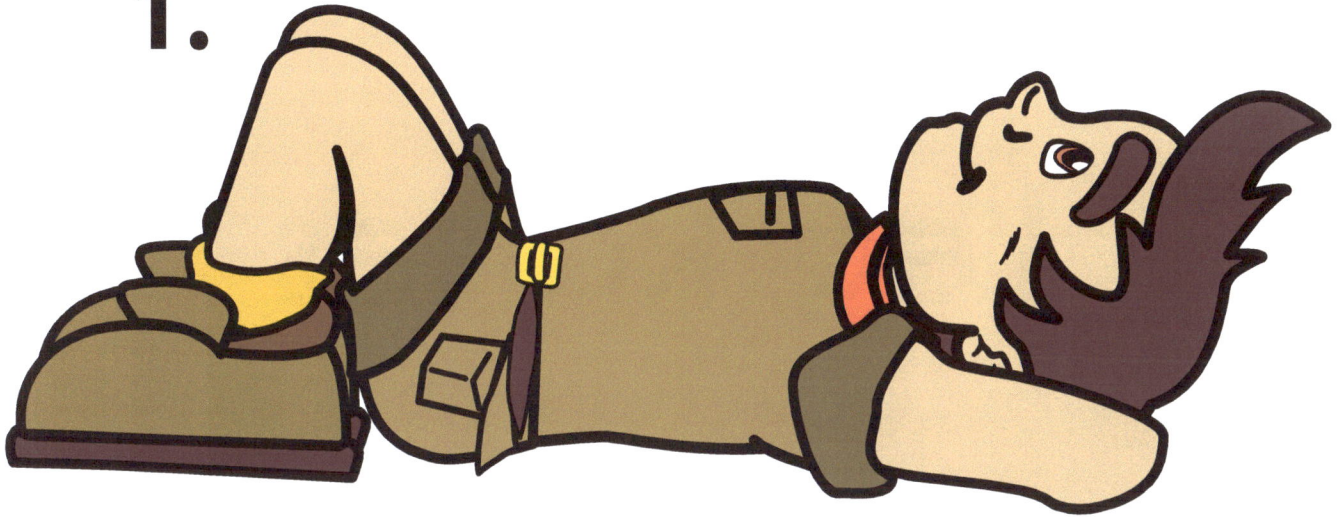

2.

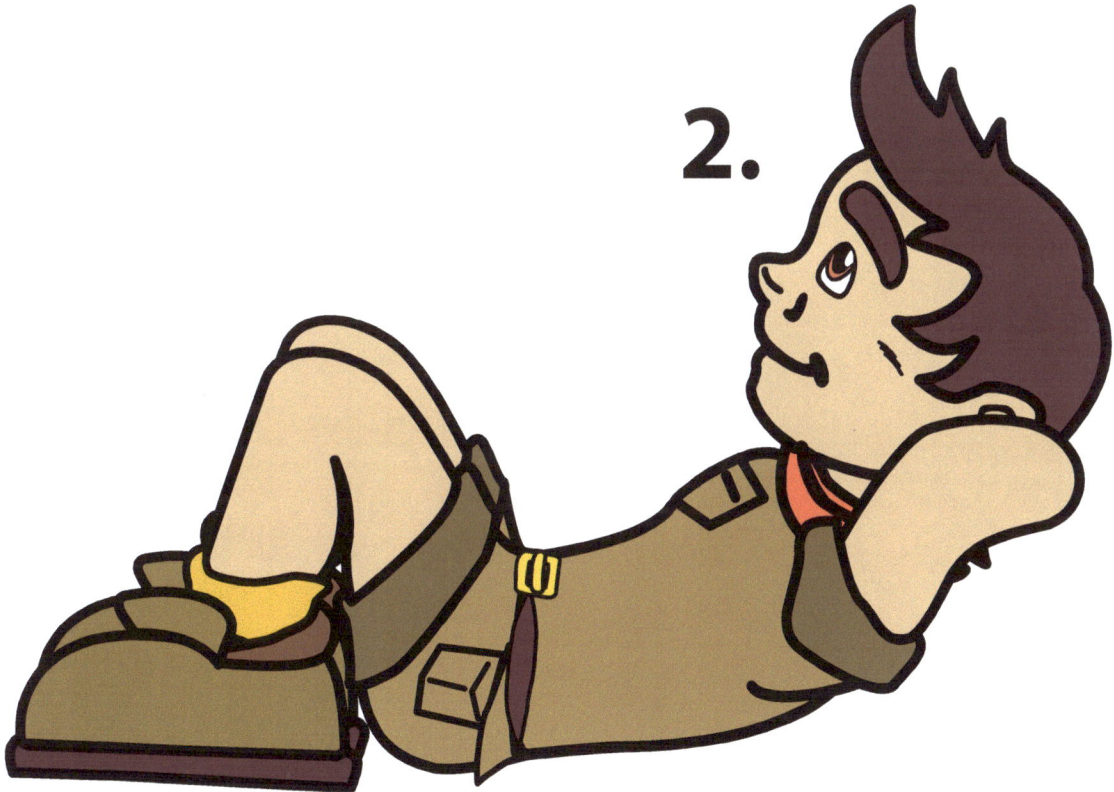

Leg Raises

Lay on your back

Keep your legs straight

Keep your elbows on the floor

Slowly bring your legs up in line with your hips

Slowly lower your legs back down

Can you do this 5 times?

1.

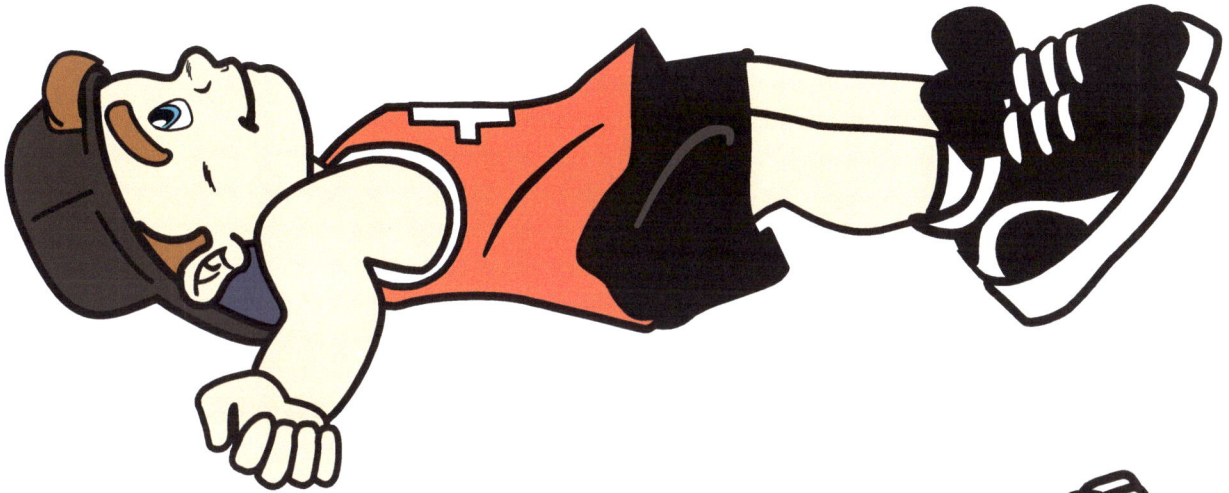

2.

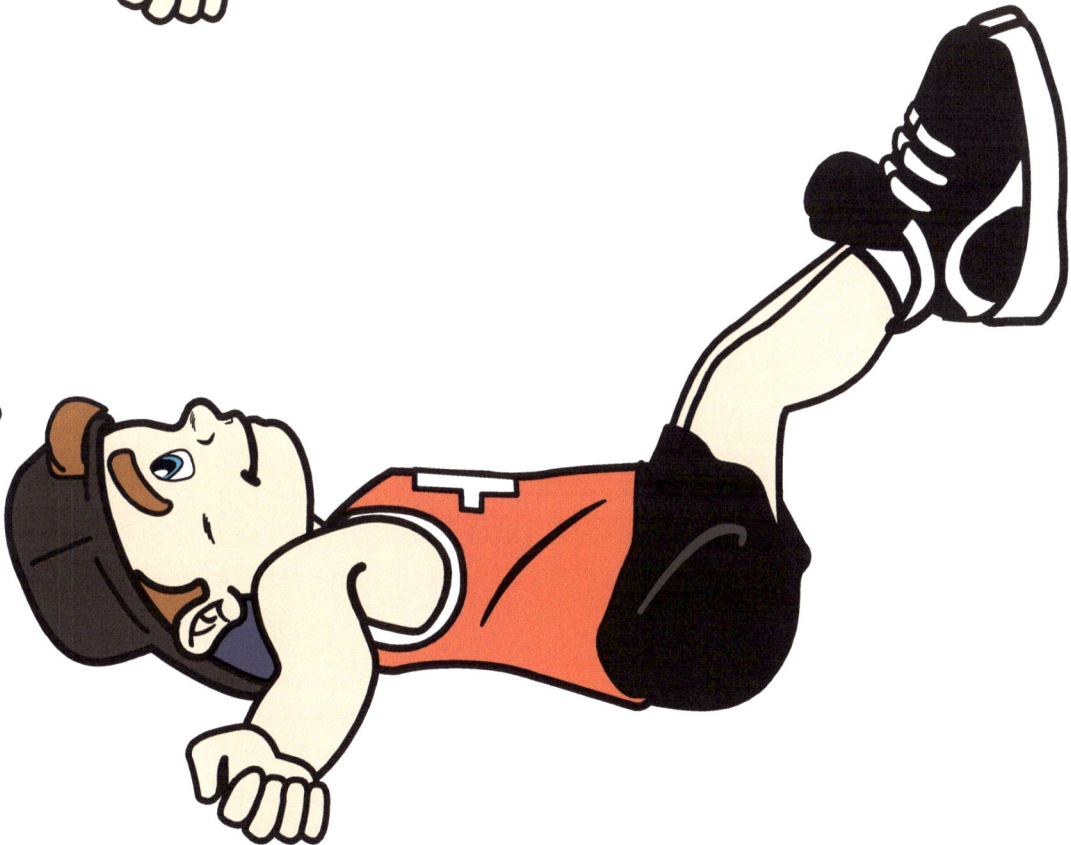

Hip Raises

Lay down on the floor

Bend your knees and face them up

Place your hands beside you

Slowly lift your hips until your body is straight

Now lower your hips back to the ground

Can you do this 5 times?

1.

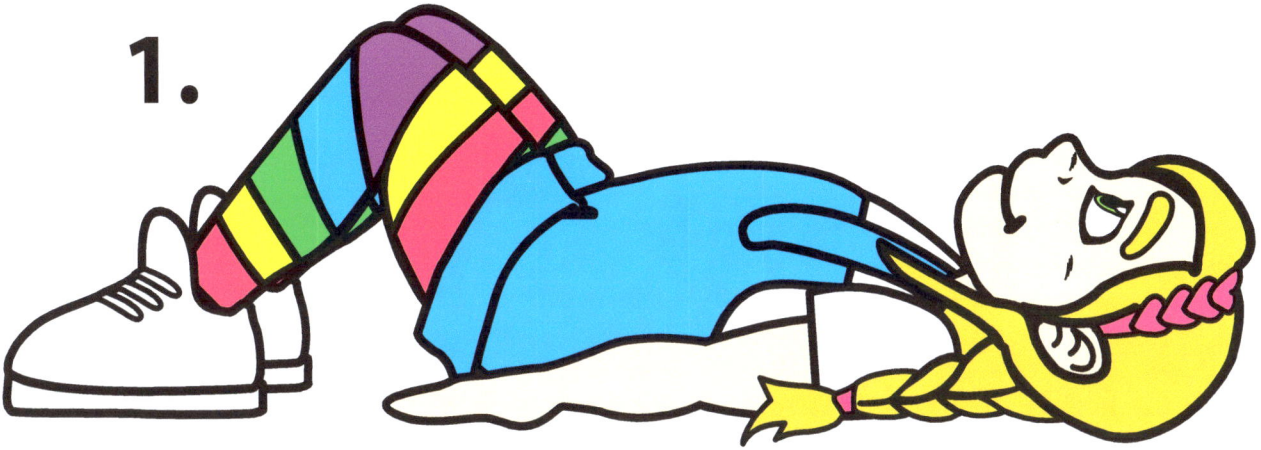

2.

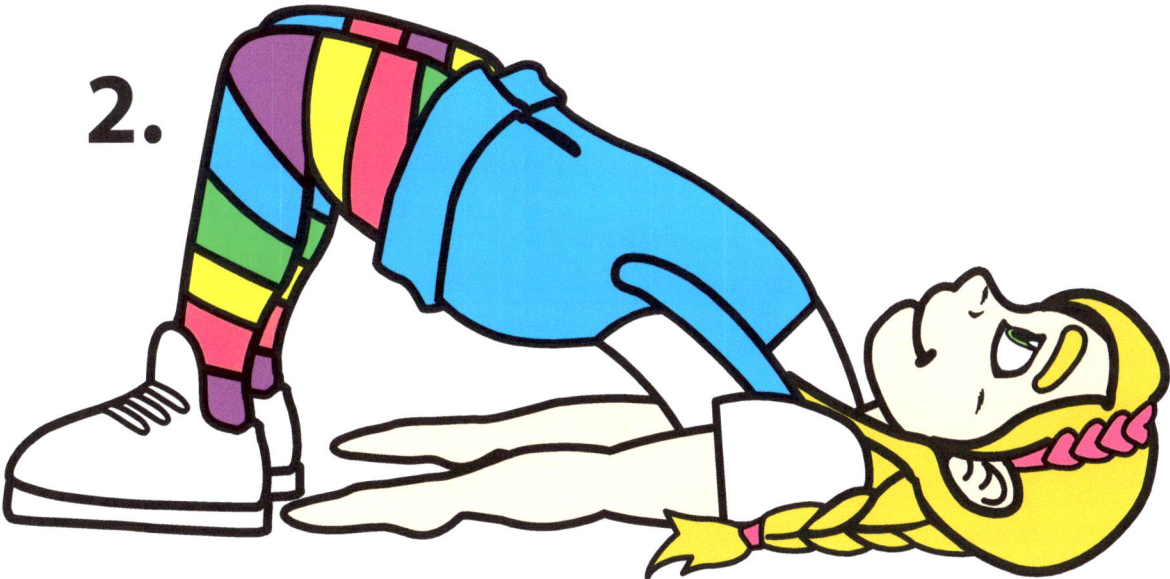

Plank Pose

Lay your stomach on the floor

Get up on your elbows and toes

Keep your back straight

Hold this for 10 seconds

Can you do this 5 times?

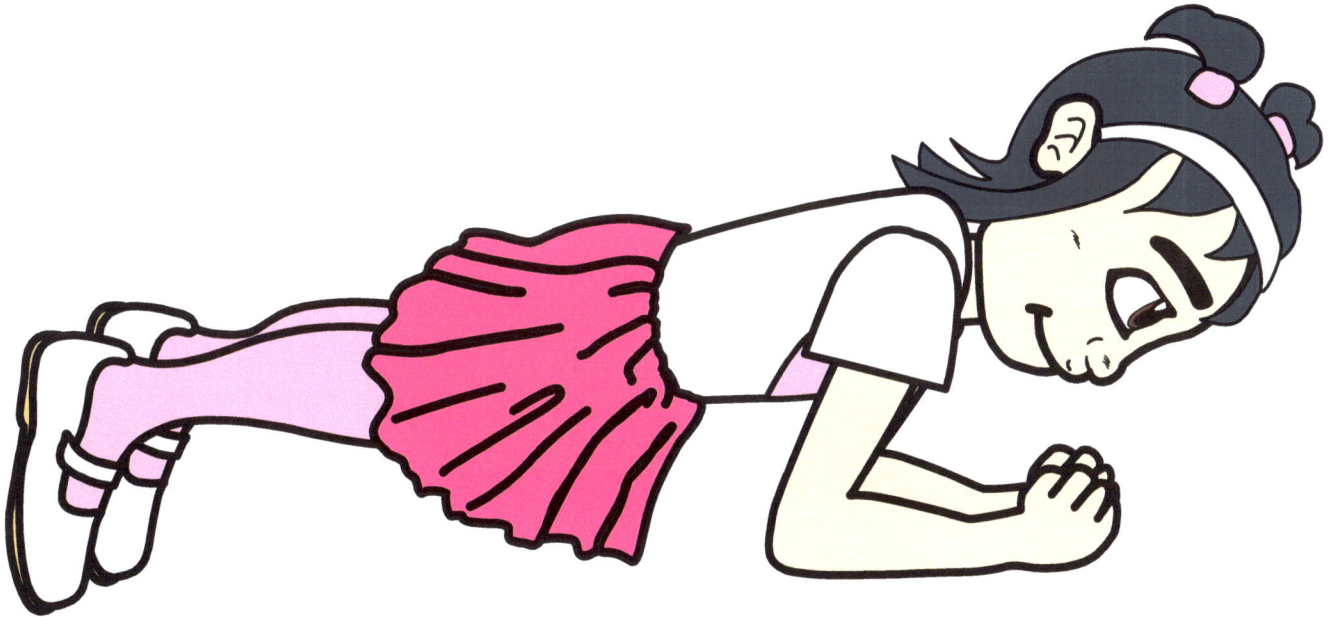

Calf Raises

Stand up straight

Keep your arms by your side

Slowly stand up on your toes

Keep your heels off the ground

Try to balance on your toes

Lower your feet back to the ground

Can you do this 5 times?

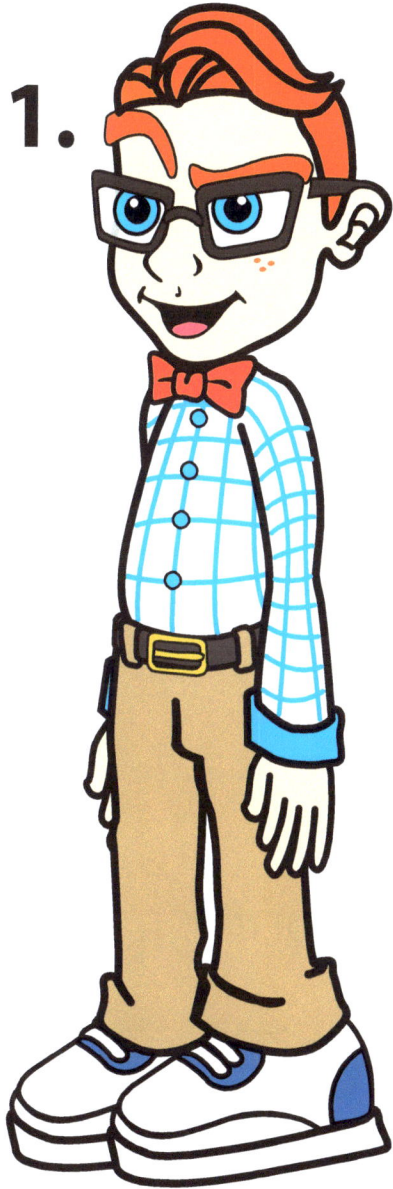

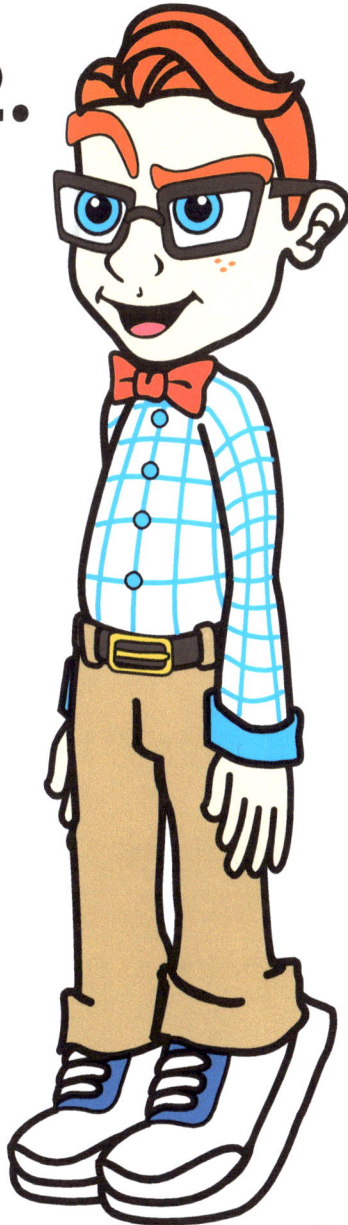

1.

2.

Body Weight   33

Squats

Stand up straight
Stand with your feet apart
Slowly lower your body
Bend your knees
Keep your back straight
Bend down only until your hip is
in line with your knees
Slowly stand back up
Can you do this 5 times?

1.

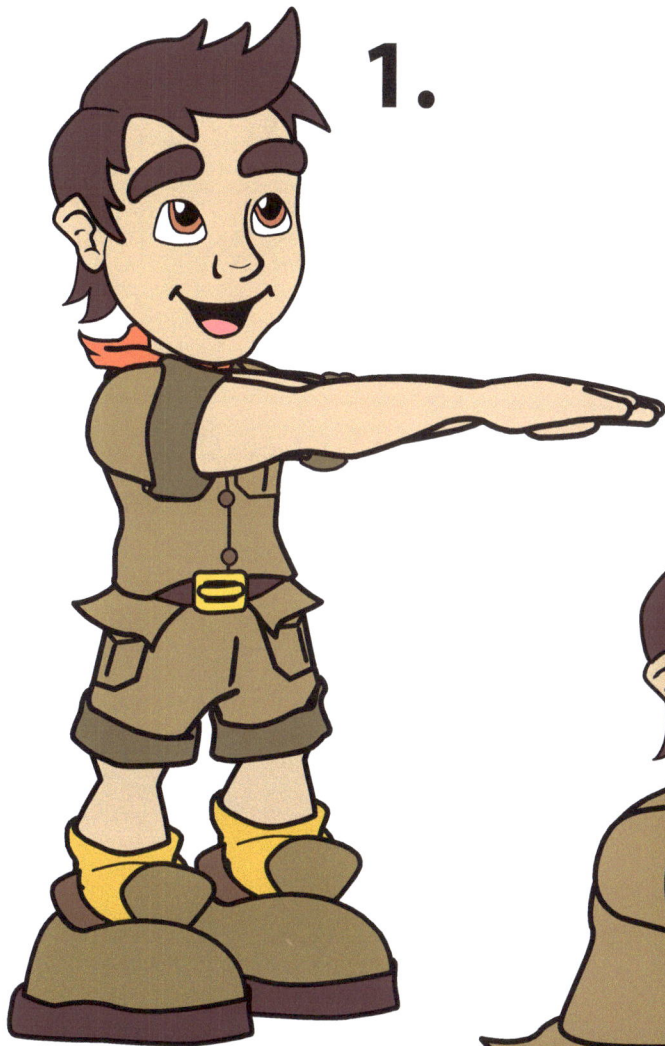

2.

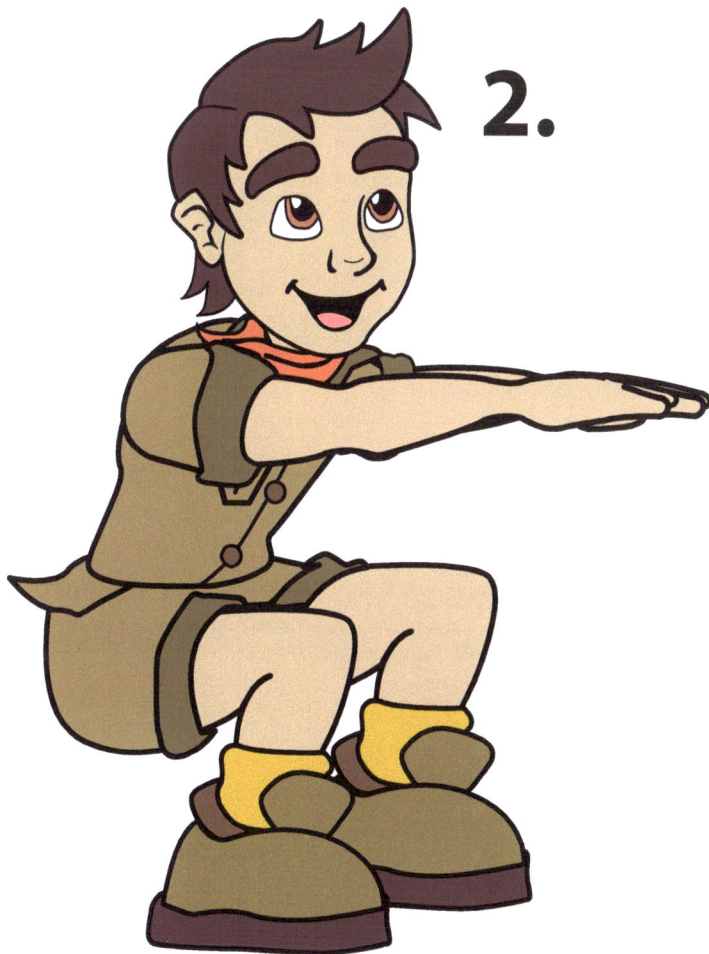

Keep an eye out for the rest of the series

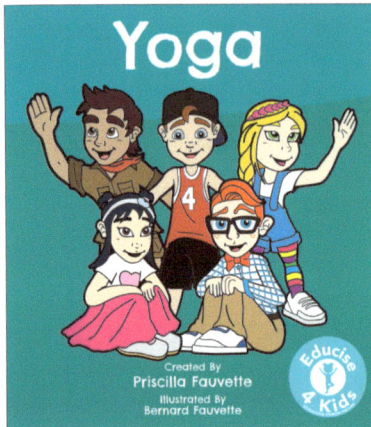

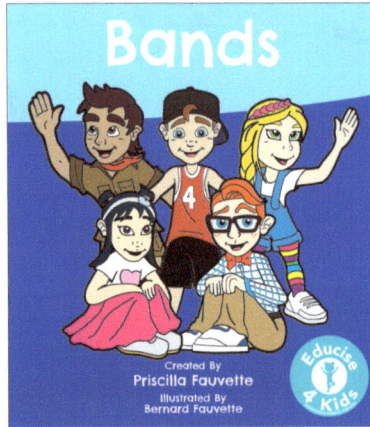

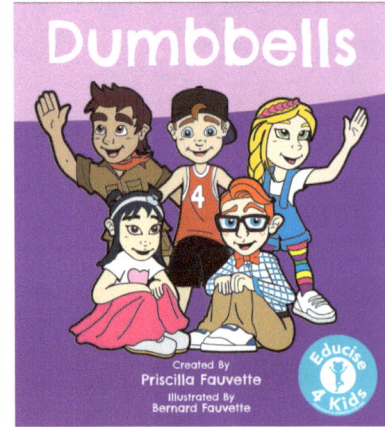

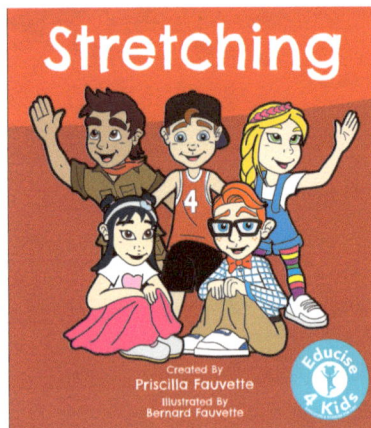

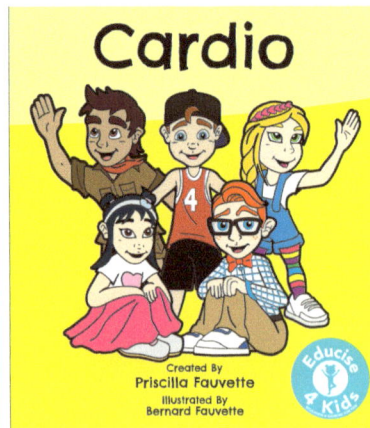

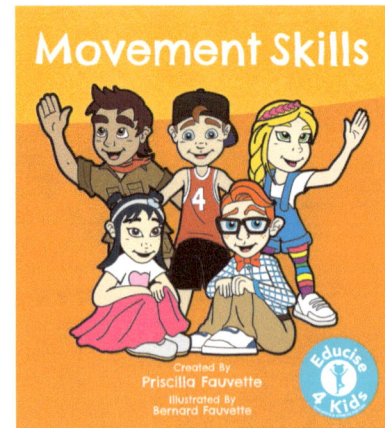

www.ingramcontent.com/pod-product-compliance
Lightning Source LLC
Chambersburg PA
CBHW061137030426
42334CB00003B/76